27 Body Transformation Habits You Can't Ignore

By Tyler Bramlett

D1026332

Although the author and publisher have made every effort to ensure that the information in this book was correct at press time, the author and publisher do not assume and hereby disclaim any liability to any party for any loss, damage, or disruption caused by errors or omissions, whether such errors or omissions result from negligence, accident, or any other cause.

This book is not intended as a substitute for the medical advice of physicians. The reader should regularly consult a physician in matters relating to his/her health and particularly with respect to any symptoms that may require diagnosis or medical attention.

The information in this book is meant to supplement, not replace, proper training. Like any sport involving speed, equipment, balance and environmental factors, the enclosed habits pose some inherent risk. The authors and publisher advise readers to take full responsibility for their safety and know their limits. Before practicing the skills described in this book, be sure that your equipment is well maintained, and do not take risks beyond your level of experience, aptitude, training, and comfort level.

Table of Contents

Introduction 1

Section 1: Daily Habits 9

Chapter 1: Drink Enough Water 11

Chapter 2: Eat Your Veggies 18

Chapter 3: Eat Protein for Breakfast 24

Chapter 4: Build A Strong Digestion 31

Chapter 5: Get Some Sleep 37

Chapter 6: Breathe Deeply 50

Chapter 7: Read A Daily Affirmation 55

Chapter 8: Walk Everyday 60

Chapter 9: Do Some Exercise 65

Chapter 10: See The Sun 70

Chapter 11: Touch The Earth 76

Chapter 12: Take A Cold Shower 81

Chapter 13: Laugh A Little 86

Chapter 14: Read Something 91

Chapter 15: Eliminate Obesogens 97

Section 2: Weekly Habits **105**

Chapter 16: Have A Cheat Meal 107

Chapter 17: Learn Something New 112

Chapter 18: Be Alone For A While 117

Chapter 19: Socialize 121

Chapter 20: Play 126

Chapter 21: Make Your Success Measureable 130

Chapter 22: Be Selfless 134

Section 3: Monthly Habits **139**

Chapter 23: Identify What Works 141

Chapter 24: Set S.M.A.R.T. Goals 145

Chapter 25: Adjust Your Plan For Success 155

Chapter 26: Create Your Own Daily Affirmation 160

Chapter 27: Do Something For Yourself 166

Conclusion 170

Introduction

Habits: Why Are They So Important?

Hello. My name is Tyler Bramlett, and I've spent the better part of a decade working with people in one-on-one settings, helping them improve their bodies and their lives. With each, new client, I find the same things to be true time and time again: No matter the client, their body, their health, and the life they were living were all a result of the habits they'd formed prior to working with me.

<u>Good or bad, habits were responsible for who they had become.</u>

I did some serious self reflecting and realized that that's all people really are - an accumulation of our habits. After I learned this, I decided that, going forward, I would focus on learning, applying and teaching people *new* habits so they could experience real and lasting change in every area of their lives.

When I began teaching my "Lifestyle Hacks" to my clients, it was easy to to see that habits are the single most-powerful way to transform a body. It was incredible seeing what consistent practice of developing new habits could do for a person.

Without fail, I could see that, as new, GOOD habits replaced people's' old BAD habits their bodies and lives were both guaranteed to change.

And that's where this book comes in. This book you're reading right now will teach you the 27 habits that I've discovered and shared with my clients. These habits will deliver to you the most powerful benefits in the shortest amount of time.

Consider this your own personal user's guide to fast-tracking your body transformation and developing the healthiest, happiest, and strongest version of yourself.

Make no mistake about it. Although this book is straightforward in its content and advice, this is not a book for people who aren't willing to make a change. If you do not change your habits, your life and your body will stay the same; however, if you develop the 27 habits I am going to teach you in this book, you will witness an incredible transformation in the way you look, feel and perform!

Get ready, because today marks the turning point in your life!!

How To Effectively Change Your Habits

Early on, when I first started teaching new habits to people I made a HUGE mistake. I was too complex in my explanations, and I expected way too much, way too fast. I would give people a giant list of things to do and expect them to do it.

And you can guess happened. My clients were resistant to all my "rules and regulations," and the good habits I was trying to teach them fell on deaf ears.

Now, I could have taken these early results personally and let my ego get in the way...but I didn't. Rather than consider this first try a failure, I simply took it as feedback that the *way* I was teaching wasn't going to work.

I went back to the drawing board, identified the most-powerful and most-important habits, and created a series of articles designed to explain each one of the habits. Each article showed them how to best apply each one, and it also showed them the quickest ways to add them into their lives for MAXIMUM benefit.

This book is a culmination of all those articles.

But I didn't stop there. Instead of just creating a book about the most-important body transformation habits that a person can use to change their lives, I went a step further and created an exact system for adding these new habits into your life. To that end, this book is divided into daily, weekly, and monthly habits, and I've even created checklists that you can use to permanently and seamlessly incorporate these 27 habits into your life, too!

All you have to do is work on adding more of these daily, weekly and monthly habits into your life and, over time, the changes will astound you. I am more than confident that, within 30 days of you consistently practicing all 27 of these habits, your life will be transformed!

Until recently, I've kept my "Lifestyle Hacks" and checklists reserved only for private clients and members of my highly-popular transformation challenges. But after witnessing the way that people's lives have improved so drastically after implementing them, I could not justify keeping these habits from the rest of the world. We all deserve to become the healthiest, happiest and strongest version of ourselves!

Please note: This is NOT another diet and exercise book designed to tell you what to eat and how to exercise. Instead, this book is dedicated to your being able to make a true and lasting life transformation. I'm going to teach you a set of new habits that are <u>guaranteed</u> to help you look, feel and perform your best.

Now that you know the idea behind these 27 habits, let's cover the best way to use this book and show you exactly how to put these habits into practice on a daily basis.

The Best Way To Use This Book

Most books like this are filled to the brim with filler text designed to fatten up the pages. But this book isn't like that. This book is straightforward and is laid out into 3, different sections. Each section has its own set of habits for you to work on. You'll find this book will be most effective if you read it using the 5 steps I've outlined below, in order.

Step One

Take the time over the next week to read through all of the 27 habits.

Step Two

Print out the Habit Forming Checklists, which you can find at, http://27habits.com/checklists and put them in a place where you will see them every day.

Step Three

Begin by doing all 5 of the Monthly Habits on your next day off. These habits will serve as the foundation for your entire month, so be sure to fill out the forms contained in the Habit Forming Checklist.

Step Four

From there, make sure you perform the following 2 weekly habits each week: (1) Kick Your Heels Up And Have A Cheat Meal AND (2) Measure Your Success. Also, pick a minimum of 1 other weekly habit, and make sure that you do that for the next 30 days. If you can manage to do all 7 Weekly habits – there is 1 habit for each day of the week - then GREAT! Be sure you check these habits off in your weekly checklist.

Step Five

Pick a minimum of 3 daily habits and focus on doing all 3 of those habits each and every day. Once you are able to do all 3 daily habits for a week, add 3 more in, and continue trying to make sure you do all 6 habits daily. It is very helpful to use the daily Habit Forming Checklists to keep track of your progress. If you prefer to jump in with both feet first and do all 15 daily habits, feel free! Just make sure not to overwhelm yourself. Being consistent is your primary goal.

Follow these EXACT 5 steps, and you will be well on your way to changing your habits and your life. Ok, now that we have the instructions out of the way, it's time for you to learn about the 27 habits!

Section 1

Daily Habits

(The Lean 15)

Your daily habits are what determine where you will be years from now. These are the 15 habits I've identified as the most powerful and important when it comes to transforming your body and your life.

Please understand that, although some of these habits may seem slightly strange and far fetched, they all serve a purpose in the grand scheme of things. If you neglect to apply them because of your beliefs or disbeliefs, you will not get the maximum benefit from this book.

If you're on the fence, all I ask is that you suspend your past belief and give these habits your sincere effort for 30 days. Once you are able to do these first 15 habits that I affectionately refer to as "The Lean Fifteen" for 30 days, you will understand their unique importance.

Important note: Many of the bad habits we've formed in life are habits are what I call silent results stoppers. If you've ever plateaued with your results, stopped losing fat, couldn't add any more reps or weight to your exercises, and experienced a crash in energy and motivation, then one of these 15 habits could be the quick fix that your body has been craving.

Let's get you started with 'The Lean Fifteen'.

Chapter 1

Our daily decisions and habits have a huge impact upon both our levels of happiness and success.

- Shawn Anchor

Daily Habit #1
Drink Enough Water

Did you know that humans can live for at least 30 days without any food [Lieberson, 2004] or that there are people like Hira Ratan Manek who claim a world record of going without eating for an incredible 400 days?

Regardless of how long anyone can go without eating, we absolutely cannot go without water for very long. The longest recorded survival without water is 14 days, with the majority of dehydration deaths occurring within only 96 hours!

Water makes up 60% or more of our total body weight and dehydration can cause a 30% decrease in performance!! [Benton, 2011]

This speaks to how important hydration is to our overall health and how important proper water consumption must be to your body. When you are dehydrated, your body actually tends to retain water and look more swollen and puffy in its fight to survive. [Wise, 2014]

Think of it like this... If you had $1000 in your bank account and you knew that there was no more money coming in, wouldn't you think twice about spending it? Wouldn't you do all you could to save it? Wouldn't you make sure that you didn't misplace any of it?

Well, this is what your body thinks when it is in a constant state of dehydration. Dehydration happens when your body loses more fluid than it takes in and can no longer perform normal functions. Becoming dehydrated will give you a soft puffy look, especially around your midsection, your feet, and your face, and it also makes your muscles tighter.

In order to fix this problem and MAXIMIZE your results, the first habit you must form is to consume a minimum of half your bodyweight (lbs) in ounces of water per day.[Wise, 2014] For example, if you weigh 150lbs you should be consuming a minimum of 75oz of water per day.

I know that sounds like a lot of water, but there's a simple way to incorporate this new habit. All you have to do is start your day with 32oz (1L) of fresh, cold water first thing in the morning. From there get yourself a 64 oz (2L) water bottle, fill it up and sip on it throughout the day.

In case you think I'm going overboard with the water, I'm not. The USDA recommends at least 91.2 ounces (2.7 liters) for adult men and women, but that recommendation can be adjusted for weight. [USDA, 2005]

In addition to quantity, the *quality* of your water can affect your recovery by supporting or breaking down your fat loss hormones. [Carey, 2010] You should be careful about the source of the water you put into your body, since many municipal water supplies contain toxic chemicals that can both reduce only your fat loss results and negatively impact your health. [Duhigg, 2009]

There are a lot of toxic substances in municipal water supplies including chromium-6, chlorine, and fluoride. [Duhigg, 2009] When these toxins enter the body, they are encapsulated by fat cells in order to protect your body.

If you simply remove toxins from your water supply, you can reduce the chances of toxin-binding fat cells forming in your body and depositing themselves in unseemly areas like your butt and thighs.

At bare minimum, consider investing in a simple, whole-house carbon filter that can remove many of the harmful chemicals from your water.

By consuming high quality water you should feel better, your body will detoxify faster and you will get better overall results by staying hydrated.

QUICK HABIT RECAP:

Drink a half of your body weight in ounces per day. Drink the purest water you can find, and if you can afford it, get a high quality water filter or have fresh spring water delivered to your house. To make sure you get enough water in throughout the day I recommend drinking 32oz. (1 liter) first thing in the morning and carrying a 64oz water bottle with you to sip throughout the day.

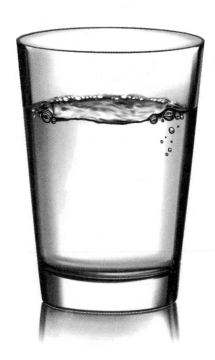

Chapter 2

Habit is habit, and not to be flung out of the window by any man, but coaxed downstairs one step at a time.

- Mark Twain

Daily Habit #2
Eat Your Veggies

Everyone knows that eating your veggies is so important, but let me ask you this question - and be honest! Do you consume the recommended 10 servings of veggies a day? [Knapton, 2014] I don't know very many people who eat the amount of vegetables that they should, every day. If I had to bet, I'd say that maybe 1 in 10,000 people eat enough veggies daily!

When you consume enough vegetables every day, your body will look and work better, and your energy levels will skyrocket. For this reason, you must form a habit of having at least 10 servings of vegetables per day. [Knapton, 2014] In case you're feeling overwhelmed, don't. Here's a simple breakdown of what constitutes a serving:

- 1 serving of raw, leafy greens = 1 cup. (This is about the size of a baseball or small fist)
- 1 serving of most other vegetables = 1 half of a cup (This is about the size of half a baseball or half a small fist)

The following methods are some of the best ways to eat your 10 servings each day.

MORE VEGGIES METHOD #1 - <u>Commit to Having a Large Salad Every, Single Day</u>

Having a large salad once daily as a meal or before your main course is a great way to boost your overall vegetable intake. It's s also a great way to prep your digestive tract before a meal.
You can keep quick and simple by using this uncomplicated and tasty recipe. Here's such a recipe that you can use (just add and subtract for flavor):

- 1 bag of your favorite greens
- One half of a large cucumber (sliced)
- 1 Carrot (sliced)
- One half of an avocado
- Olive oil and balsamic vinegar as dressing

This one salad recipe will yield an extra 5 (or more, depending on how big you make it) servings of vegetables every single day!

MORE VEGGIES METHOD #2 - ## Commit to Having a Pile of Cooked or Steamed Vegetables With Dinner

Every night for dinner, commit to having a pile even of cooked or steamed vegetables with your meal. Do this even if you had a salad earlier or if you are out to eat at your favorite restaurant. It's quite easy to add in 5 or more servings of veggies in your evening meal just by using this method.

Again, keep it simple so that you don't get frustrated. Choose vegetables that are tasty and easy to cook.

Here are my personal favorites: Brussels sprouts, broccoli, cauliflower, cabbage, carrots, spinach, kale, zucchini, squash, artichokes and asparagus.

All you have to do it steam them or lightly cook them in a pan with butter or coconut oil, and you are good to go.

MORE VEGGIES METHOD #3 - Commit to Adding Fresh Veggie Juice Into Your Daily Routine

This is perhaps my favorite method for increasing overall vegetable intake in your body specifically because it's quick to prepare, it's quick to consume, and it's nutrient-dense. Simply add 5-10 servings of vegetables into a juicer or blender and drink them down once per day. Here's basic recipe that I use that tastes great:

- 1 full stalk of celery
- One half of an apple
- On half of a cucumber
- 1-5 freshly-washed kale leaves
- Add lemon if you want more flavor

The bottom line is that you need to develop a habit of eating more vegetables. These are the best methods I have found to quickly make that happen.

QUICK HABIT RECAP:

Eat a minimum of 10 servings of vegetables per day (1 cup of raw leafy greens or ½ cup of other vegetables = 1 serving). The best ways to do this are by consuming a daily salad, adding in a pile of cooked or steamed vegetables into your evening meal, and adding in fresh juice by using a blender or a juicer.

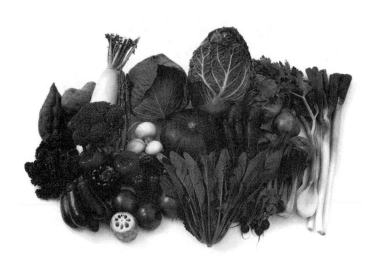

Chapter 3

Achieve success in any area of life by identifying the optimum strategies and repeating them until they become habits.

- Charles J. Givens

Daily Habit #3

Eat Protein for Breakfast

Protein is essential to getting great results. Many people have heard that they need to monitor the amount of protein they take in, but very few actually track this vital macronutrient.

The best way to make sure you get enough protein is to make a habit of eating it for breakfast.

That's right! Eating 30-50g of protein with some high quality fats and veggies for breakfast will reduce your appetite [University of Missouri-Columbia, 2013] - especially for the sweet foods - and it'll flip your fat burning switch into overdrive.

There are two reasons why this works...

REASON #1 - <u>A High-Protein Breakfast Will Level-Out Your Blood Sugar</u>

A protein-based breakfast stabilizes your blood sugar first thing in the morning. [University of Missouri-Columbia, 2013] That's EXTREMELY important when you want to lose fat. Chronically high blood sugar levels are associated with obesity, heart disease, diabetes, and more. [What Is Metabolic Syndrome, 2011]

Let me explain...

When you wake up and eat carbohydrates for breakfast, your body turns them into sugar, and your pancreas secretes the hormone insulin to get the sugar from your blood to your cells.

Much like a real estate agent, insulin's responsibility is to take the glucose (or carbs/sugar) you just ate and "house" it in a few different places. House #1 is your liver, house #2 is your muscles, and house #3 is your fat tissue.
[Bowen, 2009]

The problem with eating carbs first thing in the morning is that, unless your muscles or liver need sugar - as is the case within 60 minutes of a tough workout - the carbs will most likely choose to live in your fat cells (house #3).

Then, guess what happens when your blood sugar begins to settle down after a big spike? You crave MORE SUGAR! And you'll want it in the form of more carbs.

This whole process effectively traps you in a constant state of craving carbs and sugary foods and never lets your body go into full fat-burning mode. Skipping carbs and eating protein for breakfast is a great way to break the vicious cycle.

[University of Missouri-Columbia, 2013]

REASON #2 - <u>A High-Protein Breakfast Will Reduce Your Appetite Later In The Day</u>

A higher protein breakfast will reset your brain's responsiveness to leptin - a hormone that helps to reduce your appetite. If you always have high insulin levels in your body, you'll have less leptin [Mandal, 2014] and you will feel hungrier.

What this means is that high-protein breakfasts not only put you in fat burning mode, but they also help reduce your overall hunger. This is great news!

The habit you need to form is to eat a high protein breakfast (30-50g) generally within 60 minutes of waking. The only exception is if you follow an intermittent fasting diet in which case you'll consume protein for your first meal. If you do this, you will have better control of your blood sugar levels and will reduce your appetite and cravings for starchy and sugary carbs throughout the day.

[University of Missouri-Columbia, 2013]

NOTE: If you exercise vigorously first thing in the morning, eat your high protein breakfast directly after your workout and include carbs but minimize fat instead.

Here are a few examples of high protein breakfasts you can use:

- **Protein Mocha** - Use 30g chocolate whey protein with 16 oz coffee and 1 tablespoon of grass-fed butter. Blend in a blender and enjoy!
- **Eggs and Bacon** - Cook 2-4 eggs and 4-8oz bacon and enjoy!
- **Omelette or Scrambled Eggs** - Use 2-4 eggs along with your favorite vegetables and enjoy!
- **Meat and Nuts** - Cook 4-8oz meat (breakfast sausage works!) and eat a small handful of your favorite nuts along with it.

QUICK HABIT RECAP:

Eat 30-50g protein in the morning within 60 minutes of waking. This will regulate your blood sugar helping you to oxidize more fat for fuel and will decrease your overall appetite and cravings for starchy and sugary carbs throughout the day. If you follow an intermittent fasting diet, simply make sure your first meal is higher in protein. If you workout in the morning, lower the fat content of your meal and add in some carbs.

Chapter 4

A change in bad habits leads to change in life.

-Jenny Craig

Daily Habit #4

Build Strong Digestion

Having a healthy digestive tract is one of the most important things you can focus on if you want to boost health and vitality. In fact, did you know that 70% of your immune system comes from your digestive tract? [National Institutes of Health, 2008]

Even worse, you may not be getting the nutrients you need from your food, and a lack of nutrition could be stalling your overall results! How can this happen? Well, let's start by imagining 2 different people:

One person has excellent digestion. They can turn a rock into peanut butter, if need be. The other suffers from indigestion, constipation, and/or diarrhea. Now, imagine that both of these people eat the same meal. Are they each getting the same macro and micronutrients from the foods they eat?

Since the second person in our example above suffers from digestive issues, we need to assume that they aren't able to squeeze as much nutrition out of their meals person one with perfect digestion.

Why is this an issue? Well, let me give you the easiest explanation.

Plan and simple, our bodies are not closed chain systems. A closed chain system is one that doesn't pee, poop, sweat, etc. The only way for the people in my example above to get the exact same amount of nutrients from their foods is if their bodies were closed chain systems. [Flank, 1997]

But the human body isn't built that way. We sweat. We pee. And we poop.

Considering the fact that everyone's digestive tract and bowel movements are different, you may be absorbing less or more of the food and nutrients you eat than the person next to you is absorbing. Additionally, you might be absorbing the wrong macronutrients and/or the wrong vitamins for your body!

This is a problem because high mineral and vitamin foods tend to reduce your overall appetite while eating foods that don't have the nutrients you need tends to promote a bigger appetite!

To fix this, form the habit of *avoiding* water or other liquids right after a meal. [Nagumo, 1956] Now, I know that drinking something while and after we eat is common practice, but drinking water after a meal can dilute the digestive juices and reduce your chances of getting the maximum amount of appetite-suppressing vitamins and minerals from your diet.

Instead, give your body 60 or more minutes to digest your food before consuming liquid. In addition to this make sure you consume a minimum of one of the following sources of probiotics daily:

- Take a probiotic supplement with breakfast, every day. A probiotic supplement is one of the few supplements I take on a regular basis, and it is one that I always recommend as the #1 supplement to all of my clients.

- Consume fermented vegetables. Eating fermented veggies like, sauerkraut and kimchi can be just as effective as taking a probiotic supplement. Consume these fermented veggies as a part of your salad or with your steamed veggies.

QUICK HABIT RECAP:
Work on your digestion daily by avoiding the consumption of water or other liquids within 60 minutes of your meals <u>and</u> either take a probiotic supplement or consume a fermented food every, single day.

Chapter 5

You leave old habits behind by starting out with the thought.

'I release the need for this in my life.'

-Wayne Dyer

Daily Habit #5

Get Some Sleep

Sleep is one of the most important functions of the human body. It resets our hormones and allows our body the much needed time to repair and function optimally.

You might be thinking, *"What in the world does sleep have to do with my overall transformation?"* I get asked this question all the time.

The simple truth is that if you want to lose fat, be healthy, build muscle or be able to bring it in your workouts, then you need to form good sleep habits. Since sleep is so important, here are the habits that will help you optimize your sleep so you can look, feel and perform your best.

Sleep Habit #1:

Find Your Sleep Cycle!

First, let's myth-bust.

We constantly hear that 8 hours is the most optimum amount of sleep that a person should get each night. Unfortunately, that isn't true. You see, your body goes through different levels of sleep in a cycle.

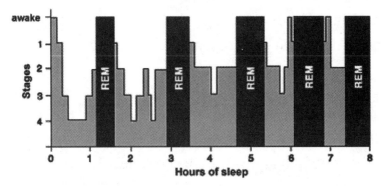

Psych Your Mind: The Sleep Cycle: What's really going on while you're catching your zzz's. (2010, September 11). Retrieved October 30, 2015.

There are periods when you're just a hair away from being awake and times when you're so deeply asleep that it would take a firecracker under your pillow to wake you.

According to the Division of Sleep Medicine at Harvard University, 'sleep cycles' tend to last from 90 to 120 minutes. If you're constantly aiming for 8 hours of sleep, you'll almost always set your alarm to go off at one of two, inopportune times: right when you're diving down into deeper stages of sleep or in the middle of coming up from those deeper stages. Either way, you'll feel "sleep drunk."

Instead of waking up ready to take on the world, you'll lay in bed wondering who glued your eyes shut, and you'll probably try to see how many times you can get away with hitting the snooze button.

This doesn't make for a very good start to your day, does it?

Instead of aiming for the age-old 8 hours, try sleeping for the following amount of hours:

DAILY MINIMUM OF SLEEP -----> 7 hours

[Rettner, 2015]

TRY TO GET THIS DAILY -----> 7.5 hours

TRY TO GET THIS ONCE A WEEK ------> 9 hours

If you do the math, you'll find that these lengths of time will ensure that you have at least four cycles of sleep per night. Now, I'm not suggesting you need to get 9 hours of sleep every night, regularly; that amount of sleep is more reserved for world-class athletes, and your body might not need that much rest.

What I am suggesting is that you get a MINIMUM of 7 hours, and that you aim for 7.5 as your norm. Then, try your best to get at least one night of 9 hours sleep per week. If you wake up feeling great, then you've nailed it. You've found your sleep cycle!

If you feel OK but not perfect, try out an 85-minute sleep cycle or a 95-minute sleep cycle instead. You'll know you've found your magic number when you wake up feeling well-rested and energized. Once you find your sleep cycle, aim for getting sleep based on that number and enjoy feeling great every day!

Sleep Habit #2 - <u>Improve Your Quality of Sleep</u>

Good sleep isn't just about quantity; it's also about quality. If you're not getting the best sleep each night even though you're sleeping at least 7.5 hours, it's time to troubleshoot.

Let's look at a few different things that can lower your sleep quality and leave you dragging the next day.

According to The Sleep Foundation, melatonin is a hormone that drives your body to sleep at night. If yours is low, you might end up counting sheep until the sun rises. There are some simple things that might affect your sleep hormone.

Those sleep factors are as follows:

- If you lack the proper amount of magnesium in your diet, you could find yourself suffering from an insomnia that you just cannot beat, no matter what you do. [Marek, 2013] Magnesium helps to regulate many of your body's daily functions at the cellular level, and you'll have a hard time producing adequate Melatonin without it.
- Light in your bedroom can reduce sleep quality dramatically. Even a dime-sized fiber optic light on the back of your knee still decreases melatonin and increases cortisol production. Research from The National Institutes of Health prove that

humans are far more sensitive to light during the night than previously understood. [Duffy and Czeisler, 2009] Bottom line: turn off the lights. Get off of your computer. And put down your phone at bedtime.

In fact, your body has photoreceptors - cells that detect light on your skin, and those photoreceptors send signals to your brain about when to turn up or down its production of melatonin. [Duffy and Czeisler, 2009]

Even small amounts of light can signal the photoreceptors to assume the sun is rising and that you want to rise with it. Melatonin likes darkness and makes us fall asleep while cortisol likes light and makes us wake up. [Duffy and Czeisler, 2009]

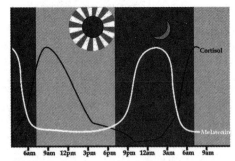

Paleo Mom. (2014, February 27). Retrieved October 30, 2015.

Knowing this, there are a few things you can do to make sure each hormone is highest at the right time.

First, get some room-darkening shades or put a dark blanket up over your windows, especially if you live in a busy city! This ensures that your melatonin levels will be at optimal levels when it's time for you to go to sleep.

Second. Reduce unwanted cortisol even further by following these guidelines:

Cortisol increases in proportion to the amount of electromagnetic frequencies (or EMF's for short) around you. Unfortunately, almost everything in our modern world produces EMF's -- light sockets, electrical outlets, your cell phone and your cell phone charger, wi-fi internet waves, radio waves, etc. [Touitou and Selmaoui, 2012]

You can't get rid of EMF's, but you can reduce them without turning into a boy in an aluminum foil bubble.

To optimize your sleep, unplug all the electronics around your bed. Get rid of your bedroom TV and replace it with an hour of reading. Reading at night increases melatonin, too. Finally, make sure your alarm clock and mobile phone are on the other side of the room while you sleep.

Sleep Habit #3 - <u>Follow Your Body's Built-In Clock</u>

Finally, do your best to go to bed when the sun goes down and get up when the sun comes up.

I realize this step may be very difficult because of your job, your family, or other obligations, so if you can't do this right now, no worries. Simply follow the above two tips and keep this tip in mind for the time when you *can* use it.

Ok...think about how we developed as a species. Did we stay up all night? Did we watch TV until right before we went to sleep? The answer to both of these questions is an absolutely NO!

Our ancient ancestors went to bed a couple hours after the sunset and woke up when the sun rose. Even in the late-1700's when life was more centered around farm life, people woke slept based on sunrise and sunset.

Why, then, are we so disconnected from nature?

Why do we stay up all night sometimes, watching goofy television shows and then complaining about being tired the entire, next day?

We do it because it's how we were raised. I don't know about you, but when I was a kid, my family watched TV shows together until right before I went to bed. When I got older, I kept the same habits. The problem is, these were bad habits!

Before moving on, I want you to know I'm not asking you to go to bed at 7pm and get up at 7am; that's completely unrealistic in this busy world. If you go to bed a few hours after the sun goes down and wake up when the sun comes up, you'll still get all the benefits of following your circadian rhythm.

Over the course of an average year, following a sunrise/sunset pattern will look something like this (depending on where you live):

- In the summer you should go to bed around 11pm and wake up with the sun.

- In the winter you should go to bed around 9:30pm and wake up with the sun.

If you can roughly follow this guideline and flow with the seasons, your sleep will improve, and the quality of your sleep will increase dramatically. Sometimes I have the opportunity of waking up naturally, and I love how great I feel on those days; however, I can't expect everyone out there to shun their jobs and lives in order to optimize their sleep.

Simply do the best you can and take advantage of the times when you can wake up naturally. Good Luck! Now, go get some sleep!

QUICK HABIT RECAP:

Sleep a minimum of 6 hours a night and aim to make 7.5 hours the bare minimum. Work on finding your own, unique sleep cycle (usually around 90 minutes) and use this when planning a good night's rest. You will know you have nailed your sleep cycle when you wake up feeling refreshed! Sleep in a dark room, and avoid electronics for a at least 30 minutes before bed. Try to go to bed within 2-3 hours of the sun going down.

Chapter 6

The only proper way to eliminate bad habits is to replace them with good ones.

-Jerome Hines

Daily Habit #6
Breathe Deeply

Breathing is arguably the most important function in the human body. [Zimmerman, 2014] As I'm sure you know, if you go without it for only a few minutes you will lose consciousness. So, how does breathing affect your overall health and results? Let's start with how you breathe.

Most people these days breathe too shallow, but if you watch any baby breathe, you'll see that it allows its abdomen to expand and contract with each breath.

I want you to take this test right now...

Place one hand on your chest and one hand on your belly. Take a huge breath in and notice which hand moves out further. If the hand on your chest puffs out while the hand on your belly stays still or even worse goes back, you are breathing in a way that your body will perceive as stressful.

If your belly moves out and your chest stays the same or slightly elevates then consider yourself a good breather.

You see, your body is governed by two entities of the central nervous system. One system is called the sympathetic nervous system. Your sympathetic nervous system regulates the 'fight or flight' feeling. The other part of your central nervous system is called the the parasympathetic nervous system. It regulates your 'rest and digest' feelings. [R. Bowen, 2006]

Chest breathing (where your belly doesn't expand) activates the sympathetic nervous system whereas belly breathing activates the parasympathetic nervous system.

This means that if you spend your days 'chest breathing' your body will constantly be in a state of mild stress. This is no good if you want to look, feel and perform your best!

Here's how you can fix this problem; make the habit of spending 5 minutes per day practicing your breathing with one hand on your chest and one on your belly until you are able to feel that your belly is doing the majority of the expanding.

Monitor yourself throughout the day by noticing if you are breathing in a relaxed manner (with your belly) or in a tense manner (with your chest). Correct yourself when you notice that you're doing it incorrectly.

Once you are breathing deeply and correctly, spend 5 minutes breathing while enjoying a walk outdoors. This one, little fix will have tremendous results. You will have more energy, and you'll feel much better.

Now that you've learned how to breathe properly, what can you do about the actual air you're breathing?

Being in polluted air is almost unavoidable, so instead of advising you to move to the forest, let's take a look at the best type of air you can breathe.

Negative ions are an electrically charged particle (atoms or molecules) that can produce profound health benefits because of the way they affect air quality. [Mann, 2009]

Both thunderstorms and the pounding of the water on the beach create negative ions that are released into the air. Those negative ions are why we "sense" the air to be fresher after a rain, after a storm, and at the beach.

So, instead of wearing a gas mask, try to put yourself in situations where the air around you is most fresh. When you can, breathe in the fresh air of the ocean, take in the crisp smell of the forest and watch how your mood and physiology shifts by simply changing the quality of the air you breathe.

If you don't live near the ocean, take a walk outside in the morning dew. Do whatever you can to reap the benefits of breathing truly fresh air!

QUICK HABIT RECAP:
The way we breathe affects our nervous system in such a way that it tells us if we are stressed or relaxed. Practice relaxed deep breathing for 5 minutes a day preferably in areas with fresh air (beaches, forests parks etc.). You can learn this style of breathing by placing one hand on your chest and one on your belly as you practice breathing into your belly while your chest minimally inflates.

Chapter 7

You gotta eat right, you gotta have healthy habits you know, and balance out your decadence with a healthy lifestyle during the day.

- Talib Kweli

Daily Habit #7

Read A Daily Affirmation

In the section on monthly habits, you will be instructed to create a daily affirmation. This daily affirmation is designed to remind you of your goals and values and it will set you up for success throughout the day.

Daily affirmations are also designed to bring you a sense of gratitude.

Being grateful is one of the key emotions that you must master in order to live a life where you can properly manage the stressors that come your way. If you want a life that you can be proud of, the ability to manage stress is critical. In fact, one of the key attributes looked at in centenarians (people who live over 100) is the fact that they are extremely good at expressing gratitude.

Many people today are always focused on what they lack, and it' understandable because our society moves at breakneck speed, nearly 24 hours a day. Do you ever remind yourself of the following?

- You still have a certain amount of weight to lose.
- You don't make enough money.
- You could use a new car.
- Your marriage isn't what you want it to be.
- You hate being single and wish you were married...

...and the list goes on and on.

The quickest way to fix a mindset that is focused on what you lack is to work yourself into a "frenzy of gratitude" right before reading your daily affirmations.

This a powerful combination of behavior that sets the pace for your day and will guide you to consistently make good choices with your habits even when you are faced with challenging situations.

Here is what you need to do: Think about all of the things you are grateful for. Say them out loud, one by one. Literally work yourself into a state where gratitude is what consumes you.

Once you've worked yourself into a "frenzy of gratitude," pull out the affirmation you have created in the Habit Forming Checklist sheets (you'll do this in the monthly habits) and read it out loud. Read it with passion, gratitude, and belief. This is a uniquely powerful way to set the pace for your whole day!

QUICK HABIT RECAP:

Work yourself into a "frenzy of gratitude" by thinking about all of the things you appreciate about your life. Then, while you are feeling deep gratitude, read out loud the daily affirmation you've prepared in the monthly habits of the Habit Forming Checklist. This is one of the best ways I know to set the tone for your day. Enjoy!

Chapter 8

A habit is something you can do without thinking-
which is why most of us have so many of them.

- Frank A. Clark

Daily Habit #8
Walk Every Day

Walking is one of my favorite exercises of all time, and there are lots of reasons why I love it so much!

- You can do it anywhere, anytime, and with zero equipment necessary.
- Walking boosts your metabolism and creates a feeling of relaxation.
- Walking promotes greater recovery and improves your immune function.
- Walking is one of the most natural movements that a human can do, and for good reason. It's how we get from place to place.

People these days walk less and less each year they're alive, and this trend is viewed as one of the major reasons for an increase in obesity and illness.

In fact, the average nomadic tribesman walks an average of 12,000 steps per day and runs in short bursts another 1,000 steps. That's 13,000 steps per day, and some estimates come in even higher at closer to 20,000 steps per day! [Karolinska Institutet, 2008]

Compare that to the average American's measly 5,117 daily steps. [Parker-Pope, 2010] Do you see where I am going with this?

Walking is one of the best overall exercises ever, and there's a good chance you're missing out on the action and the benefits!

Every day, make a habit out of doing one or all of the following 3 things to boost the amount of steps you take daily.

You will find that it will lower your stress, help you recover faster, and best of all - walking will accelerate your body transformation results!

Step #1 - <u>Start Small</u>

Take a 20-minute walk. You don't have to power-walk. A casual stroll with your family or friends will do just fine. If 20 minutes is too much, start with 10 and work your way up in 2 minutes increments each week until you've built the habit of going on a daily 30-minute walk.

Step #2 – <u>Give Yourself Reasons To Walk</u>

Park at the back of the parking lot. If you always hunt for the prime parking spot, not only will you waste time, you'll miss a valuable opportunity to take a few extra steps.

People often spend 2-4 minutes looking for the best spot instead of just parking in the back when they arrive and walking to the door faster than they could have found a spot up front. Park in the back to save time and get in some extra steps!

Step #3 - <u>Walk Off Your Calories</u>

Walk after every meal. The Chinese have a saying: *He who walks 100 steps after every meal will live to be 100.* [Furey, 2006] Walking after meals improves digestion which will help your body in numerous positive ways! [O'Connor, 2014]

There you have it! 10,000 steps a day keeps the doctor away, and it boosts your fat loss. Get out there and walk!

QUICK HABIT RECAP:

Make a habit of walking every day by going on regular 20 minute walks, parking at the back of the parking lot at stores or restaurants and taking short walks after meals. It doesn't have to be complicated, just make sure you walk every day!

Chapter 9

Curious things, habits. People themselves never knew they had them.

- Agatha Christie

Daily Habit #9
Do Some Exercise

We all know that in order to get great results you have to exercise. The problem is that there are thousands of different workout programs out there, and *none* of them seem to agree.

With all the information overload, what are you to do and who are you to believe?

Well, it's my personal philosophy that you should do some sort of exercise other than walking every single day. Now, before you freak out, let me explain what I mean by exercise.

I believe everyone should do some form of resistance training at least 3 days a week. My preference is for everyone to do some kind of higher intensity cardio training on the same schedule.

For the remaining 4 days each week, you should do something else. The goal is to move your body 7 days per week.

For the remaining 4 days, you don't have to do a vigorous workout where you break a mean sweat, and this exercise doesn't have to last for 45 minutes or longer.

Instead, do something physical for at least 10 minutes. This can be riding a bike, doing yoga, dancing, playing frisbee in the park, rolling around on the ground with your kids, gardening, or anything else that involves movement.

Try to change it up from week to week so that you're sure that you are moving your body through its full ranges of motion, every day.

This is so important because a lack of movement is one of the hardest things on your body. Jack Lalanne, the godfather of fitness said, "Move it, or lose it." Truer words have never been spoken. If you neglect to move your body every day, you eventually won't be able to move it at all.

Even patients who are bedridden are given some kind of daily movement so that their muscles don't completely atrophy while they are lying down.

QUICK HABIT RECAP:

Daily is essential in maintaining a healthy functioning body. Follow a well designed strength and cardio program 3 or more days per week and on the remaining days make sure you get at least 10 minutes of movement based exercise other than walking like riding a bike, gardening, playing with your kids etc.

Chapter 10

A long healthy life is no accident. It begins with good genes, but it also depends on good habits.

- Dan Buettner

Daily Habit #10
See The Sun

Ahh... the warm rays of the sun.

Think back to a time that you were totally relaxed, when you were outside on a park bench or relaxing on the beach bathing in the sun. Remember how relaxed you were and how amazing the sun felt on your skin? If you're able to transport yourself back to that time in your memories, you'll remember that being in the sun is a lot like being wrapped in a warm blanket. It feels great, doesn't?

So, you might wonder how something that feels so good could possibly be bad for you. Why is everyone up in arms about exposure to the sun? How could something that nourishes the earth, and provides heat and occasional relaxation, be bad for you?

Well, the answer is complicated because, while sunlight is most certainly good for you, but too much of anything is a bad thing.

Let's start with the negatives of sun overexposure. First off, the sun today is much different from the sun 1,000 years ago. As pollution increases, our ozone layer has drastically reduced and has begun to allow in harmful sun rays.

When our ozone was intact, it was possible to to get away with constant bare-skin-exposure to the sun, but that is impossible to do, now. Now, you run the risk of getting skin cancer or having some, other skin-related issue that's due to being out in the the sun for too long [Hunt, 2015].

So how do you minimize the damage from sun exposure?

Avoid going out without clothing or protection during the afternoon. For most people this will fall somewhere between 11am and 3pm. This doesn't mean you should crawl in a dark cave every afternoon.

It just means that these are some optimal hours to make sure that you *minimize* harmful sun exposure. [Price, 2015] Somewhere around 15-30 minutes is probably safer, depending on your genetics.

Secondly, all of the horror stories about skin cancer are typically related to the amount of sunburns you cumulatively have sustained in your life. [The Skin Cancer Foundation, 2015] So, more sunburns will increase your overall risk of skin cancer. [The Skin Cancer Foundation, 2015]

And herein lies the real problem. Because a lot of people are afraid of overexposure, they aren't getting enough *daily* sun exposure. If you fail to get sunlight on your skin every day, you can run into a whole host of knock-on problems.

- Without adequate exposure to the sun, your hormones won't regulate the way that they should. [Duffy and Czeisler, 2009]
- If you don't get out into the sun frequently enough each day, your circadian rhythms will be off-kilter. This means, if you want to better optimize your hormones, then you need to get some sun.
- A lack of optimal sun exposure can also lead to seasonal depression. In fact, sunlight has been proven to work as well as anti-depressants in some cases. [Duffy, Jeanne F. and Czeisler, 2009]

So, how can you use sun exposure advantageously?

Mild daily sun exposure can harmonize your body's circadian rhythm helping you sleep better and feel better...both of which and lead to better body composition. [Duffy, Jeanne F. and Czeisler, 2009]

Take a short walk first thing in the morning, letting the light hit your skin and eyes. This will help optimize your hormones right off the bat and prepare you for the day. I should mention that doing this will help to get your recommended steps right at the beginning of your day.

In addition to a morning walk, try eating your lunch outside. Again, 15-30 minutes of afternoon exposure should do more good than harm. If you can get outside later in the afternoon, even better.

The bottom line is that the sun is a lot like exercise. Getting too little or too much sun can both adversely affect your health, but if you find that happy medium, you will feel amazing, you will be healthier, your sleep will be better, and you can optimize your hormones. If your skin is light-complexioned, you might even get a good tan out if it!

QUICK HABIT RECAP:

Sun exposure is critical to optimizing our hormones and circadian rhythms. Shoot for 15 to 30 minutes of sun exposure on your skin and eyes each day, preferably avoiding the hours of 11am to 3pm.

Chapter 11

Everything you are used to, once done long enough, starts to seem natural, even though it might not be.

- Julie Smith

Daily Habit #11
Touch The Earth

Every year, information on electromagnetic frequencies or EMFs becomes more readily-accessible. If you are not familiar with what they are, let me take a moment and explain.

A bit of background, first...

A few years ago I was at a health seminar, and one of the speakers did a presentation on energy. When I write "energy," I don't mean pseudo scientific information, but rather simple facts about energy.

You see, we are all made up of energy. At the atomic level there is little that differentiates us from any other material in the universe. Energy can be seen and measured, and most importantly, it can be changed. Energy cannot be destroyed, but it *can* be changed from one state into another.

[Moskowitz, 2014]

One of the most health damaging parts of our world today are the excess EMFs floating around us all the time. These frequencies can change the way *our* energy moves and they can cause damage to our cells.

The sad truth is that most EMFs are completely unavoidable; however, there is good news!!

You see, our bodies are designed to be naturally protected from EMFs. Much like every house has a ground wire that protects its electrical system from overloading, we, too, have can ground ourselves and discharge excess EMF's.

Here's how it works...

Imagine a typical day. You wake up, take a shower, get dressed, and leave your house. While you're out, you talk on your cell phone. When you return home, you sit in front of a computer and then watch TV until it's time to go to sleep.

For most of us, from the time we wake until the time we go to bed, no part of our bodies ever touch the ground. We encapsulate your feet in rubber coated vessels that actually *prevent* energetic discharge and keep all incoming EMFs we come in contact with *within* our bodies.

So how can you get rid of these EMF's? Well...it's simple. Take off your shoes [Mercola.com, 2012] and walk on the grass for a few minutes each day.

Now I know this may sound crazy, but when your body touches the Earth - and I mean your actual skin - the earth allows you to discharge EMFs and transfer them to the Earth. How cool is that?!!

But why is it so important to discharge EMFs?

Excess EMF's can increase cortisol and insulin resistance [Hillman, 2005] which means, *more* belly fat, sugar cravings and worse overall health.

Simply walking barefoot for a few minutes a day can minimize the effects of EMFs on our bodies and help us become the most healthy, energetic version of ourselves!

QUICK HABIT RECAP:

EMFs (Electromagnetic Frequencies) are surrounding us most of the day. They have the ability to increase cortisol and insulin which means additional stress to your body. To fix this make a habit of letting your skin come in contact with the ground for just a few minutes at least once every day. When you do the the energetic bonding between your skin and the ground will dissipate the EMF's from your body and boost your overall health and vitality!

Chapter 12

The people you surround yourself with influence your behaviors, so choose friends who have healthy habits.

-Dan Buettner

Daily Habit #12
Take A Cold Shower

Cold water therapy is one of my personal favorites that I've used daily for nearly a decade.

Why does cold water therapy work and why should you hop under a cold shower, right now? It's because, being exposed to cold water increases blood flow and blood pressure [Out in the Cold, 2011] as a mechanism to keep you warm. Over time, cold showers tend to have a positive affect on blood pressure stabilization.

Cold showers also help to increase nutrient availability for your muscles which can speed up recovery times after workouts.

Cold water even has a thermogenic effect on the body. [Greenfield, 2012]

Let's break this down scientifically.

There is a type of fat cell in your body called brown fat. The formal term for brown fat is brown adipose tissue or BAT. This fat has the ability to generate heat and "burn" regular fat that's found in all the areas of our bodies that we don't want fat to exist [Greenfield, 2012]

The reason BAT burns white fat is because the white fat in our bodies are "stores" for fuel to produce heat. [Out in the Cold, 2011] If you've ever gone swimming in the cold ocean, you probably remember getting out of the water and feeling warmer. This feeling is brown fat metabolizing your surrounding fat stores for heat. [Greenfield, 2012]

There are lots of benefits from daily cold water exposure.

- An enhanced immune system.
- Higher metabolism.
- Lower and more-balanced blood sugar levels.
- Lessened inflammation after a workout...

...and the list goes on.

In my opinion, cold showers are one of the most important habits that you can quickly incorporate to increase your overall health.

I don't want you to go for a swim in the ocean or pack yourself with ice, but you add a short 2-5 minute rinse at end of your shower. Once you get used to it, you will feel invigorated!

QUICK HABIT RECAP:

Exposing yourself to cold water has so many benefits I could write an entire book on the subject. Add in 2-5 minutes of exposure to cold water at the end of your shower on a daily basis and reap these amazing health and vitality benefits!

Chapter 13

Consciousness is a phase of mental life which arises in connection with the formation of new habits. When habit is formed, consciousness only interferes to spoil our performance.

- William Ralph Inge

Daily Habit #13
Laugh A Little

Laughing is one of the best things you can do for your body.

When you genuinely laugh out loud, your body gets flooded with endorphins. [Gorman, 2011] Many cancer centers are now even recommending exposure to laughter for their patients. [Gorman, 2011]

Just google laughing and cancer and you will see lots of amazing stories.

Knowing these facts, why aren't we laughing more. Why do many people stop thinking that things are funny and shut down?

I believe the reason is a result of 2 things.

HUMOR KILLER #1 - <u>The Media</u>

When you sit down today and watch your local news, what do you see?

Are there heroic stories, comical happenings, and happy endings? Not really, right? Instead, the images that are constantly placed before you include lots of crime, violence, poverty, death and plenty of other negative things.

This is a huge issue because the media is making us believe that the world is a dark and evil place. I'm all for being well-informed; however, I choose to limit my exposure to negative media. Because of this, I notice a profound positive effect on my mood.

Even with work and family-related challenges, I am an exceptionally happy person...and that's because I love to laugh and do it often.

If you can't find a way to laugh, try eliminating or limiting exposure to negative media. Watch something that makes you feel good. Dare to laugh!

Eventually, your stress levels will lessen, and you will be able to enjoy life more.

HUMOR KILLER #2 - <u>YOU</u>

My friends and family all know me as someone who rarely has a filter on my thoughts and opinions. I try my best to move through life in a great, joyful haze. I try to find the humor in everything!

In fact, just days before writing this I came down with a really bad case of the stomach flu. After throwing up all night long I looked over to my wife and said, "You know, people pay good money for a cleanse this good." We both looked at each other and laughed.

Many people these days take themselves and situations too seriously. Our culture disapproves of public laughter and prohibits us from truly embracing humor. So, stop taking yourself so seriously and enjoy your life with laughter!

The way I am able to do this is to let go of regimented seriousness and instead, I try to see the world like my child does. I'm sure you can remember a little of what it was like to be a kid.

Children don't care what anyone thinks about their actions. Just watch any 5 year old. Children that age live free of almost any social conformities.

To get into the childlike and free mindset, try to put yourself into situations that make you laugh.

- Hang out with a funny friend.
- Watch a funny show.
- Turn on some stand up comedy that you like.
- Listen to a funny podcast or audio program and try enjoy it!

By habitually laughing each and every day, you will boost your immune system, flood your body with endorphins and reduce stress!

QUICK HABIT RECAP:

Laughing daily can boost your immune system, flood your body with happy hormones and give you a greater sense of relaxation and ease in your life. Laugh daily by avoiding too much negative media exposure, taking yourself less seriously and putting yourself into more humorous situations.

Chapter 14

Habits are the daughters of action, but then they nurse their mother, and produce daughters after her image, but far more beautiful and prosperous.

- Jeremy Taylor

Daily Habit #14
Read Something

There's a quotation I heard years ago by Harry S. Truman, and it stuck with me. He said, "Not all readers are leaders, but all leaders are readers."

I've learned, over time, that this quotation is true. Reading is a powerful form of self-education that expands your mind and lets you experience life more fully. The most successful and intelligent people I have ever met are all avid readers.

Sadly, reading for pleasure is becoming less-popular.

Did you know that between 33 and 36 percent of young people exiting high school now are predicted to never read another book again? [Stack Exchange, 2012]

Book readers by age

% who have read a book in whole or in part in the past 12 months

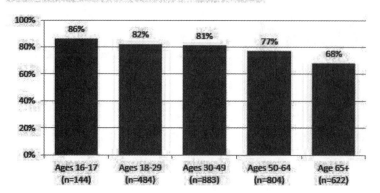

Source: Pew Research Center's Internet & American Life Reading Habits Survey, November 16-December 21, 2011. N=2,986 respondents age 16 and older. Interviews were conducted in English and Spanish and on landline and cells. The margin of error for the sample is +/- 2 percentage points.

Rainie, L., Zickuhr, K., Purcell, K., Madden, M., & Brenner, J. (2012, April 4). Part 2: The general reading habits of Americans. Retrieved October 30, 2015.

And did you know that the percentage of the population that reads on a regular basis is on a steady decline? [Stack Exchange, 2012]

Having unlimited data at our fingertips is making it harder for us to keep our attention on paper. Even with all of these facts, it's still true that reading will always to be the best way to exercise your brain.

I recommend at least 15 minutes of reading per day. Keep it simple to start.

- Find a book that interests you.
- Set a timer to help you know when your time has ended.
- When that timer goes off, find a good place to stop, mark where you stopped reading, and call it a day.

Over time those 15 minutes will become a refuge for you...an escape from this crazy world.

Remember, readers are leaders!

QUICK HABIT RECAP:

All of the smartest and most successful people are readers. Develop the habit of reading for 15 minutes a day by choosing a book that interests you and setting a timer for 15 minutes. Once the timer is up mark where you left off and wait until tomorrow. Over time you will learn to love the time you spend reading and you will keep your mind sharp into old age.

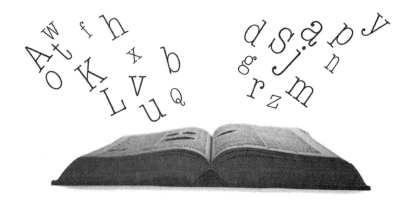

Chapter 15

I think if you stop bad habits, and you stop long enough, you develop good habits.

- Jordan Knight

Daily Habit #15
Eliminate Obesogens

I don't want to be an alarmist, but there are toxins in your home that you *need* to avoid.

These toxins destroy your health and stall fat loss. The worst thing about them is that they are found in many of your household items.

These household toxins are called obesogens. Do you see the root word "obese" in obesogen? If you do, the word itself should give you a clue into what they do.

Quite plainly, obesogens are a class of chemical compounds that disrupt the normal growth and metabolism of lipids. Molecules that include lipids are fats, steroids, fat-soluble vitamins, and others.

[Holtcamp, 2012]

In other words, when you ingest obesogens via whatever mode, - skin, air or via your food - your body tends to store *more* body fat and make it harder for you to lose the fat you're storing!

[Holtcamp, 2012]

So, what the heck can we do about obesogens?

Unfortunately, it's impossible to eliminate 100% of obesogens. So, in order to reduce their effects, we should eliminate as much of their use as we possibly can.

Here is a list of the **top 5 things** you should eliminate from your household in order to minimize unnecessary exposure to obesogens:

Stop Drinking or Eating Off Of Plastics

That's right. Plastic. Plastic is one of the biggest players in the obesogen game. Instead of using plastic containers and zip lock bags, try using glass cups and storage containers as often as you can.

Avoid Store Bought Air Fresheners

Most air fresheners contain obesogens. Instead of chemical-ridden generic air fresheners, try using natural fresheners that you can get from your local health food store. Better yet, light a candle or buy a diffuser and use organic essential oils to scent your home.

Avoid Packaged Or Processed Foods

You may have already tackled this one, but you should know that most packaged and processed foods contain sufficiently high amounts of obesogens. The less your food is processed, the more likely you will be to avoid obesogens. As much as you can, buy certified organic groceries. This should help you to minimize obesogen contact!

Ditch The Non Stick Pans

Although extremely convenient, non stick pans release poisonous chemicals into the air and into your food that are known to be harmful to both the environment and to you! [Holtcamp, 2012] Do your best to trade up to cast iron or stainless steel.

Stay Away From Chemical House Cleaners

Chemical house cleaners contain absurdly high amounts of obesogens. It's time for you to choose whether you want shiny, spot-free windows or rapid fat loss?

Most local health food stores sell natural cleaning supplies that make avoiding obesogens and other harmful chemicals a lot more convenient. They also do a pretty good job of cleaning, too.

Try replacing your cleaners a little bit at time. Find what you like.

Remember, all you have to do is make changes one step at a time. Don't get overwhelmed by all of this information. Though it might feel like it's a lot to process, your only job is to take a little bit of action, consistently, every day.

Focus on one of the categories I've shared with you in this section at a time until you have replaced all of your toxic household products with the obesogen-free versions. Good luck!

QUICK HABIT RECAP:

Obesogens are chemicals found in many common household items. They mess with your lipid metabolism and hormones and the result is a decrease in your health and fat gain.Make a habit of avoiding the 5 main obesogens above including; eating or drinking off of plastic materials, store bought air fresheners, stay away from packaged or processed foods, do not use non stick pans that contain teflon and do not use chemical based house cleaners.

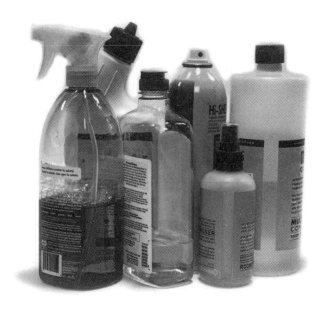

Section 2

Weekly Habits

(One for Each Day of the Week)

This is the weekly one habits section, and there is one for each day of the week. Though these habits are performed less often than the daily ones, they all play an integral part in you changing your body and your life.

Unlike the daily habits, most of the weekly habits are very enjoyable and are very easy to do. Since there are seven habits, all you have to do is perform just 1 habit each day of the week, and you are good :)

Start out by doing the following two habits as a priority.

1. Kick up your heels and have a cheat meal, and...
2. Measure your success.

Once you are firm on these two, pick one or more additional habits to focus on and become consistent doing.

Over time, you will develop a consistent practice of all seven habits, which will help you look, feel and perform your absolute best.

Alright, let's introduce you to the 7 weekly habits...

Chapter 16

Your net worth is usually determined by what remains after your bad habits are subtracted from your good ones.

- Benjamin Franklin

Weekly Habit #1
Have a Cheat Meal

While I am a stickler for maintaining a good nutrition program, I am also a huge advocate of taking a meal (or a day if you're fairly lean) to eat whatever you want.

The reason for this is because the quickest way to give up on a nutrition program, is to deprive yourself of certain foods for too long. If you're worried about the effects of a cheat day, trust me, a measly meal or 12 hour window of eating some tasty foods will not affect your results as long as you are following good nutrition the rest of the week.

Even on a cheat meal, or a cheat day, I have a few rules to help you minimize overall damage. Follow these rules before and during your cheat meal for best results.

- Start your day off with a high-protein meal just like you do on all other days.
- Make sure you still consume enough protein throughout the day.
- Drink lots of extra fluids throughout the day before your meals. Remember: Don't drink anything right after you eat!
- Consume hot herbal teas such as green tea or yerba mate tea in order to help digestion and increase your metabolic rate.
- Be sure to try and exercise or stay active in order for your body to handle all of the excess carbs you consume.
- Reduce your fat intake when consuming a high carb meal.
- Don't eat something if you feel you are having an allergic or uncomfortable reaction from it. Common foods sensitivities are wheat, dairy, legumes, shellfish, eggs, etc.
- Don't feel guilty. Be happy and enjoy your day!

QUICK HABIT RECAP:

Having a cheat meal (or day if you are lean) once per week where you enjoy your favorite foods is a good idea to keep you motivated to stick to a good diet. Follow the tips above to reduce any damage caused from cheat days.

Chapter 17

You've got bad eating habit if you use a grocery cart in 7-Eleven.

- Dennis Miller

Weekly Habit #2
Learn Something New

Even though this book is about incorporating new habits, I'm sure at some point you will come to think they're too hard to fully apply. This is because, learning new things is hard, plain and simple.

This means that it's harder to learn newer things, like all these new habits. Brain science is the key to habit-strengthening.

Dr. Donald Hebb, a PHD researcher in the fields of neuroscience once said, "Nerves that fire together wire together." When applied to the fitness industry, we've interpreted his saying to mean that the more you do something, the better you get at it.

Think about it like this: If you put a hose at the top of a hill and turn it on, within 5 minutes, there will be dozens - perhaps even hundreds! - of different water trails flowing down the hill. This represents the way the synapses in the brain work when you learn something new.

If you keep learning over the course of a week, a month, or even years, those "tracks" will eventually turn into deep grooves, which represents deeply-ingrained neural pathways.

What does this have to do forming better habits?

A lot.

The longer you spend creating bad exercise, nutrition and lifestyle habits, the more likely you are to have a hard time eliminating those bad habits. Quite literally, you may be trying to undo 30, 40 or 50 years of mental conditioning...so it might be hard at first.

Now, I don't mean to discourage you, but I want you to know the truth. I also want to show you a way increase your neuroplasticity and kiss your old habits goodbye much more quickly.

Here's how:
In order to relearn, you have to actually practice learning.

What you're going to do is learn something new. I don't care if it's physical or mental. Whatever it is, dedicate yourself to it. This will unlock areas of your brain that have never been accessed before.

Here are just a few recommendations of things you can learn:

- Learn a new movement or sport.
- Do things the opposite way you usually do them. For example, put your left shoe on first, brush your teeth left handed, write left handed, etc.
- Try a new, healthy recipe, every week. You will surprise yourself with the foods you didn't know you liked.
- Watch a documentary, and then have a discussion about it with someone.
- Take a class or an online course in something that interests you.
- Try a new outdoor activity.

The point is simple. When you learn new things, your brain will open up to new possibilities, and the more options your brain has, the less likely you are to get stuck in a rut of any kind.

Once a week, devote 30 minutes to learning something new.

It can be anything you want. Focus on that one thing for as long as you need, and practice it each week. Or you can change it every week. Try it out and get ready to surprise yourself with the fun results you're going to see!

QUICK HABIT RECAP:

When you learn new things your brain rewires itself to be more receptive to developing new habits. Spend 30 minutes each week learning to do something new. It can be anything you want, the more creative the better. You can work on one thing for months or change every week.

Chapter 18

Vices are often habits rather than passions.

- Antoine Rivarol

Weekly Habit #3
Be Alone
for A While

Today, some people consider it a badge of honor to not take care of themselves. You hear people talk about how they only sleep 4 hours, work 2 jobs and spend all their free time with their family and friends.

The problem with this is that when you are constantly distracted with work and other people, you tend to neglect yourself. Eventually, this can result in you forgetting who you are and what you love to do.

I'm not recommending that you prioritize your needs over your family, but I *am* suggesting that everyone, including the busiest people in the world, take a little time for themselves.

Carve out an hour or more a week to do something that you love to do. <u>And to do it alone.</u>

It's important you do this alone so that you can reflect on your values and connect with yourself. Doing this regularly will help you develop a profound sense of self-awareness that not many other people possess.

Don't forget that if you have responsibilities like a spouse or children, you must work together to make sure they get an equal opportunity to do the same. Doing this for each other will cultivated a greater level of respect as well as a deeper connection between yourself and your partner if you have one.

The difference is astounding!

QUICK HABIT RECAP:

Carve out an hour once per week to do something that you love to do alone. It is important that you do it alone as the purpose of this habit is to develop a sense of self awareness you cannot develop any other way. Make sure to return the favor to your spouse or family members by allowing them the same time for themselves each week.

Chapter 19

Motivation is what gets you started. Habit is what keeps you going.

- Jim Ryun

Weekly Habit #4
Socialize

Just like we need time to ourselves, we also need time with our family and friends. This is important because, as humans, we are social by nature. If we avoid social contact for extended periods of time because of depression or anxiety, we become disconnected from both ourselves and from others.

[Dworkin-McDaniel, 2011]

There are indeed differing personality types. Some people need varying types of socializing, and some require more than others, but humans are meant for relationships.

We were designed to deeply enjoy our friends and family in different kinds of environments, But, our busy lives often keep us away from physical social settings. Instead, we turn too often to our TVs, iPads, and mobile phones.

To fix this and reap the benefit of socialization, set aside a minimum of one hour each week to spend quality time with your family or friends. It is important that you choose a good setting and make sure that you avoid all distractions.

That means you should put away your phone and all other digital devices. Nothing spoils a social setting more than digital devices. The following are some good examples of ways to socialize with your family and friends:

- Eat at a restaurant that has outdoor patio and let everyone know that there will be **no** cell phones allowed.
- Go to a park and enjoy some outdoor time with your family.
- Have a BBQ outside!
- Do a group activity like roller skating or cooking a meal.

At first this may seem a little difficult, especially if you have children, but over time, socializing will grow into a fun and pleasurable time for you to connect with those you love.

Regardless of what activities you choose to do, take 60 minutes out of the week to avoid technology and be physically present with your family and friends.

QUICK HABIT RECAP:

As humans, we are social creatures. As social creatures, we thrive on regular, meaningful human interaction. Set aside 60 minutes or more each week, away from technology (including TV, computers and mobile phones) to socialize with your family and friends. Some great social settings are parks, beaches, restaurants and backyard BBQ's.

Chapter 20

Everything you are used to, once done long enough, starts to seem natural, even though it might not be.

- Julie Smith

Weekly Habit #5
Play

Do you ever just look at children? Do you watch them play on the playground? You know how much fun they have? If not, next time you are around children take notice of how joyful they are when just moving freely around any space.

Where did we lose this?

Didn't we use to play like that?

The truth is, we value education so highly, that we have forgotten how enjoy just moving around. Unfortunately this isn't the way we were designed to operate at our best.

So what can we do to retrieve this playful state of being? Simple. Join the children!

I'm not suggesting that you go running up and down the slides or that you try to compete with little ones for their space on the playground. What

I am recommending is that you set aside 30 minutes each week to get outside and play a little.

This can serve as a great way to get fresh air, exercise, sun exposure, learn new movements, socialize and get your feet on the earth. You can actually incorporate many of your new habits into this one habit if you want to!

Here are some ideas of things you can do that are playful, fun and can actually boost your fat-loss results:

- Rock-climbing
- Paddle-boarding
- Walking
- Hiking
- Surfing
- Soccer
- Baseball
- Capture the Flag
- Frisbee
- Flying a kite
- Playing catch
- Walking your dogs

You can do pretty much anything that you have fun doing!

QUICK HABIT RECAP:

Playing like a child (especially outdoors) is key t a healthy and happy life. Set aside 30 minutes a week to simply play. You can do anything that you love to do and this can serve as a great way to accomplish many of the other habits at the same time.

Chapter 21

H is for Habit, winners make a habit of doing the things losers don't want to do.

- Lucas Remmerswaal

Weekly Habit #6
Make Your Success Measurable

Thought leader and bestselling author Robin Sharma said, "What gets measured gets improved." That is a very appropriate quotation at this point in the book.

Since the goal of this book is to teach you how to transform you body and life by mastering new habits, it stands to reason that one of the habits you need to do each and every week is set aside time to measure your success, reflect on your goals, and take careful note of how you are progressing at incorporating your new habits into your life.

Set aside 10 minutes each week to ask yourself the following questions so that you can measure your success:

- Are you consistently performing the *daily* habits that you are working on developing? If yes, then great. If not, then what do you need to do to make those habits more consistent?
- Have you performed each of the *weekly* habits you are working on this week? If yes, then great. If not, then what do you need to do to make those habits more consistent?
- Have you been following the monthly plan you created in the Habit Forming Checklist for your SMART Goal? If yes, then great. If not, then you'll need to determine what adjustments gets to be made to your plan in order to make it work better?

Once you honestly reflect on what you have accomplished for the week, tweak your daily affirmation to reflect any changes you've made that will help you be more consistent. You are forming new habits and the work to following the plan you've laid out to achieve your goals is important.

QUICK HABIT RECAP:

Set aside 10 minutes to reflect upon the successes and failures you've had each week. Are you staying consistent with your daily and weekly habits? Are you following the monthly plan to achieve your goal that you created in the Habit Forming Checklist? If yes, then great if no, what do you need to do to make those habits more consistent? Alter your daily affirmation to reflect any changes you make to help you be more consistent.

Chapter 22

So much of what we do every single day is the result of habits we have formed over time.

- Joyce Meyer

Weekly Habit #7
Be Selfless

There are few things more satisfying than performing a truly selfless act for someone else. The joy and gratitude that the other person experiences when you do something nice for them has the ability to make you a better person.

Additionally, the ripple effect of someone remembering the nice act that you did for them will likely affect more people over time. Try to think back to a time when actually someone did something nice for you or for another person another person else without expecting anything in return.

Maybe you've watched videos on YouTube of people giving to the poor, paying it forward, or helping the homeless. It felt good to watch acts of kindness towards others, didn't it? It made you feels a happier and more-fulfilled that day, too, didn't it?

The most important part of this section is to encourage you to make more selfless decisions on behalf of others. When you perform a selfless act, you cannot expect anything in return.

No thank you.
No forgiveness.
No acknowledgement.

You must give honestly and completely. This will do more for you in the depths of your soul than you can fully understand until you do it.

Whatever you decide to do, does not have to be expensive. It doesn't have to be done publicly. But maybe it will cost money. And maybe it will be done in public. It's really your choice.

You could just give a nice pep talk. You might give someone who is having a bad day a hug. Maybe you'll decide to buy a cup of coffee for a coworker.

If you have bridges to mend in your family or other relationships, surprise them by doing something nice for them.

For the most impactful results, do this weekly for someone you don't know...someone who is a complete stranger to you.

During an interview I conducted, I learned of an interesting way to selflessly give back that you can try.

Go to a local coffeehouse and purchase a gift card for whatever amount you want. Give it to the person taking orders and tell them to use the card for the next people until it runs out and walk away.

If you want, you can sit outside with your coffee and watch as people smile from the surprise.

QUICK HABIT RECAP:

Perform one truly selfless act each week for another person. Do not expect anything in return, not even a thank you or a smile. For best results, do something for someone you do not know and make it anonymous if possible.

Section 3

Monthly Habits

(The Foundation for Habit Building)

This section contains five essential monthly habits that serve as the foundation for all the other habits in this book.

Unlike the other sections, where the habits are relatively straightforward, four of these habits involve your critical thinking and creativity.

<u>You must do all five of these habits for the rest of this book to work.</u>

By doing all five of these habits once per month, you will develop a deep sense of self-awareness, purpose and direction that few other people have.

These habits will serve as your roadmap to yourself and guide you to succeed with this book.

Make sure you have your Habit Forming Checklist pages printed out (you can find them at http://27habits.com/checklists)as you will be actively participating for the first 4 monthly habits.

Let's jump right in and lay the foundation!

Chapter 23

Play reaches the habits most needed for intellectual growth.

- Bruno Bettelheim

Monthly Habit #1
Identify What Works

One of the most challenging things for people to do is to look at themselves objectively. We all have preconceived beliefs about ourselves and of our self worth. The good news is that your perception of yourself isn't your complete reality. It's simply an intellectual projection of your own, current physical being.

This concept was really challenging for me to put onto paper in a way that makes sense. I guess what I am trying to tell you is that you are who you are in this moment, right now. But there is another "you" in the future...someone you're working to become.

The only way you can make a change is to accept where you are currently and then identify where you want to go in life. It is only after you do this that you will be able to plan to change yourself and head in the direction of your dreams and goals.

Establish where you are, objectively. As you do, you'll automatically see what is not working, as well.

Bringing It All Together:

Make sure you print out your Monthly Forms (there are six of them), and fill out Form 1 and 2 right now to assist you in establishing where you're at and what's keeping you from becoming the best version of yourself!

Chapter 24

Habits change into character.

-Ovid

Monthly Habit #2
Set S.M.A.R.T. Goals

I'm gonna lay it on the line here and say that there's a good chance you want to look better naked, right? There's no shame in that. In fact, when people come to work with me privately, I first try to get them to set some goals and expectations.

Typically they'll beat around the bush saying they only want to improve their health and fitness but, ultimately it boils down to their dissatisfaction with the current state of their body.

Identifying your primary goal is crucial to getting optimal results, because you can never reach a destination if you don't know its location. Wherever you are right now, I want you to take a moment to think about what it is that you really want to accomplish with your body.

Is it a great body fat percentage, between 16-18% for females or 8-10% for males? Would you like to compete in a sport again? Do you want your husband or wife to call you hot, buff or sexy again?

Once you have an idea of how you want to look, feel, or perform. I want you to write the following statement down on paper and read it several times each day.

Here it is: *You can achieve anything you want as long as you know where you are going and what steps you need to take to get there.*

After you identify your goals, all you have to do is stay the course, keep doing what's working and eliminate anything that isn't working. You will eventually arrive at your destination!

Let's imagine a hypothetical scenario. Let's say you want to lose 10% body fat. This is a good goal, because if you lose 10% body fat, you will be a brand new person.

Take that goal, write it down, and read it every day. Internalize it until you feel like it's the only thing is going to happen, like it's become part of your being.

You need to research how other people have done this so that you can be clear on what works, but for now, let's pretend you're going to work out with kettlebells and cross training coupled with a low-sugar, low-processed diet with moderate to high protein (just like you're already doing).

You have a plan now. All you have to to do is follow it, make some tweaks if necessary, and improve on the program. Make it yours! Let's look at the best way achieve these goals.

Set S.M.A.R.T. Goals

Each letter in S.M.A.R.T. stands for Specific, Measurable, Attainable, Relevant and Time Bound. Let's break down each letter, now:

Specific

The more specific your goal is, the better. If you want to lose 10% body fat which statement is more powerful; "I want to lose 10% body fat" or "I will lose 10% body fat by January 1st 2013 as registered on an ultrasound body fat scanner using a 7 point test."

The bottom line is this: The more specific the goal the more likely you are to achieve it. Be exact!

Measurable

You want to be able to measure all your progress. Imagine if you had said you wanted to lose 10 lbs this year. This is not very specific goal, but that's not why it's a problem.

The problem is this: If you have a body transformation goals, you should focus on something more measurable. To that end, percentages don't lie. If you have a low body fat percentage and good relative muscle mass, you will look good in a bathing suit.

If you you are unspecific and set out to lose 10 pounds and you also lose all muscle along the way, guess what? You still won't be happy.

Make sure that you know what you are going to measure and how you are going to measure it. It will also help you to have milestones to mark your progress.

Attainable

We already talked about this a little. Your goal needs to be something feasible.

That written, you should aim high, and your goal should give you butterflies. Your goal should also make you feel good thinking about it. You need to know your capabilities, and you should set your goals just a little higher so that you shoot for something amazing.

It sounds difficult, but I see people reach goals all the time that they never thought they'd reach. You can do this!

Relevant

You won't finish something that is unimportant to you. This is especially important when setting financial goals.

If you tie your goals to a number (i.e., I want to make $5,000 more this year), then you also assign some sort of significance to that number.

What does the $5,000 represent? Is it a vacation you want to take? Are you saving it? Is it a down payment on a new car?

If the reason isn't strong enough, you're going to struggle attaining that goal, so make sure you are setting goals that tap into your deepest passions and make sure you have your reasons why written down so that you always know why you're working towards this goal.

Time Bound

No goal is complete without a deadline.

I recommend working backwards from your goal date and setting mini goals. For example, if you weigh 150 lbs with 30% body fat and want to weigh 135 lbs with 20% body fat in one year, your mini goals should look something like this:

Start - 150 lbs, 30% body fat
3mo - 146 lbs, 28% body fat
6mo - 142 lbs, 25% body fat
9mo - 138 lbs, 22% body fat
12mo - Finish at 135 lbs, 20% body fat

At first glance, these mini goals look tiny in comparison to a year, but that's why they're so important.

If all you focused on was losing four pounds and two percent body fat every 12 weeks, you would end with amazing results after the year. Small steps every day are the true building blocks of sustainable results.

DO THIS RIGHT NOW!!

Take out a piece of paper and write down *"I will set a S.M.A.R.T. goal specific to what I want, write it down, and put it in a place where I will see it daily. I will do this right now."*

You have set your first S.M.A.R.T. goal.

All you have to do now is take some time to come up with your S.M.A.R.T. goals.

Bringing It All Together:

Now that you understand S.M.A.R.T Goals, go back to your Monthly Forms (there are six of them), and fill out Form 3. This will help you establish your goals and create a roadmap for how you will achieve them!

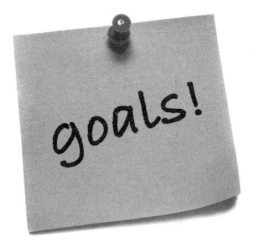

Chapter 25

Good habits are worth being fanatical about.

- John Irving

Monthly Habit #3
Adjust Your Plan for Success

Your goals are like water. They flow with you on the endless journey of life. In order for you to make a real and lasting change, you shouldn't become married to a particular method of achieving your goals.

The most successful people on the planet set specific goals, and they make plans to achieve those goals just like you. The only difference between the extremely successful and everyone else is their ability to adjust and adapt as they move towards their goals.

You see, when most people are met with roadblocks, they get frustrated and end up quitting. They tell themselves that their plan didn't work and reconcile themselves to a life of blameless mediocrity. But, instead of seeing failure as total defeat or as a reason to give up, what if you used failure as a way to analyze whether your plans to achieve your goals are working.

What if you used failure as an education?

Thomas Edison once said after failing over 10,000 times to invent the lightbulb, "I didn't fail 10,000 times, I found 10,000 ways not to make the lightbulb."

His perseverance is the reason you and I can flip a switch and light a room.

The reason why I am telling you this is because if you really want to achieve your goals, then planning and adjusting that plan monthly or even sooner is the best way to get you there!

Pull out your Monthly Habit Forms right now, and follow along to the questions as you use your 30 Day SMART goal to set or adjust your plan. Make sure you are always on the right path for success!

Remember, <u>there is no failure</u>. There is only knowledge of what worked for you and what did not.

__Bringing It All Together__:

Now that you are clear that you get to make adjustments as needed, go to the Monthly Forms (there are six of them), and fill out forms 4 and 5 to further specify your current plan. Adjusting is a big part of the process so don't feel bad if you establish a plan and fail to execute it.

Michelangelo said, "The greater danger for most of us lies not in setting our aim too high and falling short; but in setting our aim too low, and achieving our mark."

Chapter 26

Successful people are simply those with successful habits

- Brian Tracy

Monthly Habit #4
Create Your Own Daily Affirmation

When your goal is body transformation, how important is your mindset? The truth is...what is going on in your mind is highly underestimated.

Your brain is the heavy-hitter in this game - especially when it comes to optimizing your results.

Once I heard a story about a woman who taped a piece of paper over the display of her scale. The paper showed her goal weight of 132 lbs, which was about ten pounds less than her current weight.

Every day she stepped on the scale, looked down at the fake number, pretended it was real, threw up her arms in excitement and exclaimed, "Yes! I did it!"

The tale ended 60 days later.

She'd repeated the same ritual, daily. Without any significant nutrition or exercise changes, she peeled away the paper, stepped on the scale and found that she weighed 132 lbs!

I don't know if the story is true or not, but it's a compelling idea to think about what your subconscious can do to your results.

Consider the following two people, decide who will succeed:

Person 1

This person wakes up every morning and thinks, "Today is the best day ever! I've got my food planned, I can't wait to work out. I know with every fiber of my being that I'm on the right track. Fat loss, here I come!"

OR...

Person 2

This person wakes up every morning and thinks, "I'm so tired! This diet is hard and these workouts are tough. Maybe I'll skip today. Besides, I don't even know if this program will work. Nothing ever goes right for me."

Okay. I may have made it way too easy to choose the winner of this mindset game, but you need to understand how important self-talk is.

If you say you're tired, you'll be tired. If you say you hate working out, you'll hate working out. Whether or not you think you are person 1 or 2 right now, consider creating a daily affirmation that you can read to yourself every day.

Put it beside your bed and read it first thing every morning. It'll motivate you and put you in the right mindset.

This has been instrumental for me in my life.

I started silently reading a small paragraph on an index card several years ago and have since evolved into listening to a 5-minute speech that I recorded about where I want to be in the future.

Here are some guidelines for your daily affirmation:

- Write in the future. Instead of writing, "In 45 days I will weigh less," write, "It's November 11th and I'm 11 pounds lighter. The choices I've made over the last 50 days have led me to this huge success!"
- Give yourself as much clarity as you possibly can. Include details about how it'll feel to accomplish your goal, who you'll tell, the clothes you'll wear and any other details that will make your goal feel more real every time you read it.
- End it with a statement of gratitude. Try saying something like, "I am so grateful for where I am in my life, and I'm excited for what I know I can do. Thank you!"

Here's a full example:

"It's November 11th, and I'm 11 pounds lighter. My skinny jeans fit again and I feel the best I've felt since I was 19! The choices I've made over the last 50 days have led me to this huge success and I am so grateful for where I am in my life. I'm excited for what I know I can do! Thank you!"

Bringing It All Together:

Now that you understand daily affirmations, go to the Monthly Forms (there are six of them), and fill out form 6 to assist you in creating your affirmation for the next 30 days.

Chapter 27

"Your beliefs become your thoughts,
Your Thoughts become your words,
Your words become your actions,
Your actions become your habits,
Your habits become your values,
Your values become your destiny."
-Mahatma Gandhi

Monthly Habit #5
Do Something for Yourself

Self care is perhaps one of the most neglected areas of many peoples lives. When you don't take the time to care for yourself, you won't ever be able to care for others.

By doing something to take care of yourself at least once a month, you will improve your health, your happiness, and the way your body feels and looks.

Here's just a few of the things you could consider doing to take care of yourself:

- Get a massage.
- Go to a day spa and spend the day soaking in their tubs or visiting their sauna.
- Go see a chiropractor.

- Get rolfed (seriously...you have to try this!)
- See a therapist you can comfortably talk to.
- Go to a weekend retreat for some much needed rest and relaxation.
- Schedule some extra time to sleep in with no distractions.
- Take your spouse or family on a trip to the beach and relax in the sun

There are many more things I could put on this list, but you understand my point. The bottom line is to do something for YOU. Do something that you know will make you feel like a million bucks and will rejuvenate your body and mind.
Don't forget, if you have a spouse or significant other it's a great idea to help them out by encouraging them to take care of themselves at least once a month as well. The benefits to your relationship will be tangible and will grow as time passes.

Bringing It All Together:

Now that you know the importance of taking care of yourself, put this book down right now and schedule in some time to do something nice for yourself.

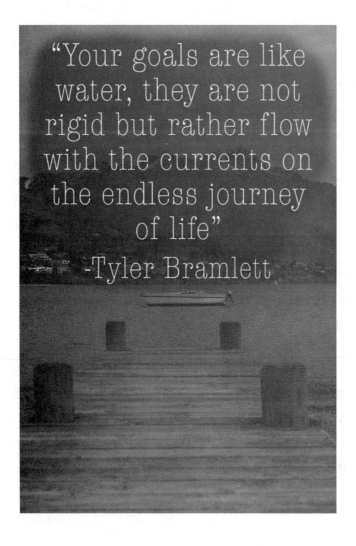

"Your goals are like water, they are not rigid but rather flow with the currents on the endless journey of life"
-Tyler Bramlett

Conclusion

Change your habits:
By the inch it's a cinch. By the yard, it's hard!

The real key to you becoming a happier and healthier version of you who looks, feels and performs their best is in changing your habits. This is not an overnight endeavor however and the single most important thing is for you to be consistent and persistent.

This book and the accompanying Habit Forming Checklists will guide you through developing the 27 Body Transformation Habits that will change your life for the better. If you apply the information in this book, I can honestly and confidently guarantee that you will feel better than you ever thought you could feel!

As a final note...never give up on working to improve yourself. Always keep moving forward towards your goals, and when you get stuck (and you *will* get stuck), don't get frustrated but rather learn the lessons that life is trying to teach you and then find a way to continue on your path to becoming the greatest version of yourself.

Remember, I'm here to help if you need me. :)

Tyler J. Bramlett
AKA - The Garage Warrior

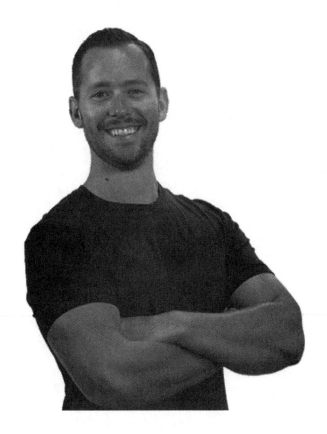

References

1. Benton, David. "Dehydration Influences Mood and Cognition: A Plausible Hypothesis?" Http://www.ncbi.nlm.nih.gov. US National Library of Medicine National Institutes of Health, 11 May 2011. Web. 7 Oct. 2015. http://www.ncbi.nlm.nih.gov/pmc/articles/PMC3257694/.

2. Bruso, Jessica. "The Serving Size for Dark Green, Leafy Vegetables." Http://healthyeating.sfgate.com. SF Gate. Web. 7 Oct. 2015. http://healthyeating.sfgate.com/serving-size-dark-green-leafy-vegetables-2655.html.

3. Duhigg, Charles. "That Tap Water Is Legal but May Be Unhealthy." Http://www.nytimes.com. The New York Times, 13 Dec. 2009. Web. 7 Oct. 2015. http://www.nytimes.com/2009/12/17/us/17water.html?_r=0.

4. Dworkin-McDaniel, Norine. "Touching Makes You Healthier." Http://www.cnn.com. CNN, 5 Jan. 2011. Web. 7 Oct. 2015. http://www.cnn.com/2011/HEALTH/01/05/touching.makes.you.healthier.health/.

5. Flank, Lenny. "Does Evolution Violate the Laws of Thermodynamics?" Http://www.huecotanks.com. 1997. Web. 7 Oct. 2015. http://www.huecotanks.com/debunk/thermo.htm.

6. Gorman, James. "Scientists Hint at Why Laughter Feels So Good." Http://www.nytimes.com. The New York Times, 13 Sept. 2011. Web. 7 Oct. 2015. http://www.nytimes.com/2011/09/14/science/14laughter.html.

7. Hillman, Donald. "Exposure to Electrical and Magnetic Fields (EMF) Linked to Neuroendocrine Stress Syndrome: Increased Cardiovascular Disease, Diabetes and Cancer." Http://www.electricalpollution.com. Shocking News, 1 Nov. 2005. Web. 7 Oct. 2015. http://www.electricalpollution.com/documents/Hillman/ShockingNewsv8-112005.pdf.

8. Knapton, Sarah. "Healthy Diet Means 10 Portions of Fruit and Vegetables per Day, Not Five." Http://www.telegraph.co.uk. The Telegraph, 31 Mar. 2014. Web. 7 Oct. 2015. http://www.telegraph.co.uk/news/science/science-news/10735633/Healthy-diet-means- 10-portions-of-fruit-and-vegetables-per-day-not-five.html.

9. "Laughter Therapy." Http://www.cancercenter.com. Cancer Treatment Centers of America. Web. 7 Oct. 2015. http://www.cancercenter.com/treatments/laughter-therapy/.

10. Lieberson, Alan D. "How Long Can a Person Survive without Food?" Http://www.scientificamerican.com. Scientific America, 8 Oct. 2004. Web. 7 Nov. 2015. http://www.scientificamerican.com/article/how-long-can-a-person-sur/.

11. Mandal, Dr. Ananya. "What Does Leptin Do?" Http://www.news-medical.net. News Medi- cal, 13 Jan. 2014. Web. 7 Oct. 2015. http://www.news-medical.net/health/What-Does-Leptin-Do.aspx.

12. Nagumo, Masako. "Gastrointestinal Regulation of Water and Its Effect on Food Intake and Rate of Digestion." American Physiological Society 188.327-331 (1956). Http://ajplegacy.physiology.org. American Physiological Society. Web. 7 Oct. 2015. http://ajplegacy.physiology.org/content/188/2/327.article-info.

13. "Out in the Cold." Http://www.health.harvard.edu. Harvard Health Publications, 2011. Web. 7 Oct. 2015. http://www.health.harvard.edu/staying-healthy/out-in-the-cold.

14. Parker-Pope, Tara. "The Pedometer Test: Americans Take Fewer Steps." Http://well.blogs.nytimes.com. The New York Times, 19 Oct. 2010. Web. 7 Oct. 2015. http://well.blogs.nytimes.com/2010/10/19/the-pedometer-test-americans-take-fewer-ste ps/?_r=0.

15. Price, Dr. Dzung. "Building Better Bones – What Women In Their 50s Can Do To Prevent Bone Loss (Osteoporosis)?" Http://beyondgoodhealthclinics.com.au. Beyond Good Health: Holistic Medical Clinics, 13 July 2015. Web. 7 Oct. 2015. http://beyondgoodhealthclinics.com.au/category/hormon al-balancing/.

16. Rettner, Rachael. "How Much Sleep Should You Get? New Recommendations Released." Http://www.livescience.com. Livescience, 3 Feb. 2015. Web. 7 Oct. 2015. http://www.livescience.com/49676-new-sleep-recommendations.html.

17. "The Ultimate Antioxidant: Fight Premature Aging for Free." Http://articles.mercola.com. Mercola.com, 4 Nov. 2012. Web. 7 Oct. 2015. http://articles.mercola.com/sites/articles/archive/2012/11 /04/why-does-walking-barefoot-on-the-earth-make-you-feel-better.aspx.

18. "What Is a Serving?" Http://www.heart.org. The American Heart Association, 18 Feb. 2015. Web. 7 Oct. 2015. http://www.heart.org/HEARTORG/Caregiver/Replenish/ WhatisaServing/What-is-a-Servin g_UCM_301838_Article.jsp.

19. "What Is Metabolic Syndrome?"
Http://www.nhlbi.nih.gov. National Heart, Lung and
Blood Institute, 3 Nov. 2011. Web. 7 Oct. 2015.
http://www.nhlbi.nih.gov/health/health-topics/topics/ms.

20. Wise, Abigail. "7 Sneaky Reasons You're Bloated."
Http://www.huffingtonpost.com. The Huffington Post, 10
June 2014. Web. 7 Oct. 2015.
http://www.huffingtonpost.com/2014/06/10/bloating_n_
5439816.html.

21. "Dietary Reference Intakes For Water, Potassium,
Sodium, Chloride, and Sulfate"
http://www.nal.usda.gov/ The National Academies
Press, 2005. The Institute of Medicine of The National
Academies for the USDA.
http://www.nal.usda.gov/fnic/DRI/DRI_Water/water_ful
l_report.pdf

22. Carey, Adam. "Water CAN Make You Fat: How
Chemicals in Drink Can Trigger Weight Gain And
Fertility Problems" http://www.dailymail.co.uk. Web.
The Daily Mail, 27 March 2010.
http://www.dailymail.co.uk/health/article-
1261203/How-water-CAN-make-fat-chemicals-drink-
trigger-weight-gain-fertility-problems.html.

23. "Protein Rich Breakfast Helps Curb Appetite
Throughout the Morning" http://www.sciencedaily.com.
Web. Science Daily for the University of Missouri-
Columbia, 14 Nov. 2013.
http://www.sciencedaily.com/releases/2013/11/1311141
02528.htm.

24. "Consuming high-protein breakfasts helps women
maintain glucose control, study finds"
http://www.sciencedaily.com Web. Science Daily for the
University of Missouri-Columbia, 29 April, 2014.

http://www.sciencedaily.com/releases/2014/04/1404291
62110.htm.

25. Doyle, Marek. "Help Me Sleep: Magnesium Is The
    Secret For Sleep Problems."
    http://www.huffingtonpost.co.uk/ The Huffington Post,
    22 May, 2013. Web. 22 July, 2013.
    http://www.huffingtonpost.co.uk/marek-doyle/help-me-
    sleep-magnesium-secret-to-sleep-
    problems_b_3311795.html

26. "Allergy and the Gastrointestinal System"
    http://www.ncbi.nlm.nih.gov. Web. US National Library
    of Medicine National Institutes of Health, Sept 2008.
    http://www.ncbi.nlm.nih.gov/pmc/articles/PMC2515351
    /.

27. Bowen, R. "Physiologic Effects of Insulin"
    http://www.vivo.colostate.edu/. Web. Colorado State
    University, 1 Aug, 2009.
    http://www.vivo.colostate.edu/hbooks/pathphys/endocri
    ne/pancreas/insulin_phys.html.

28. "Natural Patterns of Sleep."
    http://healthysleep.med.harvard.edu. Web. The Division
    of Sleep Medicine, Harvard University, 18 Dec. 2007.
    http://healthysleep.med.harvard.edu/healthy/science/wha
    t/sleep-patterns-rem-nrem.

29. Duffy, Jeanne F. and Czeisler, Charles A. "Effect of
    Light on Human Circadian Physiology." Published by
    PubMedCentral 4 June, 2009. Web. 1 June, 2010.
    http://www.ncbi.nlm.nih.gov/pmc/articles/PMC2717723

30. Touitou, Yvan and Selmaoui, Brahim. "The Effects of
    Extremely Low-Frequency Magnetic Fields on
    Melatonin and Cortisol, Two Marker Rhythms of the
    Circadian System." Web. Pubished by PubMedCentral
    14 December, 2012

http://www.ncbi.nlm.nih.gov/pmc/articles/PMC3553569
/

31. Zimmerman, Kim Ann. "Respiratory System: Facts, Functions, and Diseases." http://www.livescience.com. Web. Livescience. 1 Oct. 2014. http://www.livescience.com/22616-respiratory-system.html.

32. Bowen, R. "The Enteric Nervous System." http://www.vivo.colostate.edu/. Web. Colorado State University. 24 June, 2006. http://www.vivo.colostate.edu/hbooks/pathphys/digestion/basics/gi_nervous.html.

33. Mann, Denise. "Negative Ions Create Positive Vibes." http://www.webmd.com. Web. Web MD, 6 May, 2002. http://www.webmd.com/balance/features/negative-ions-create-positive-vibes.

34. Karolinska Institutet. "Regular Walking Protects The Masai -- Who Eat High Fat Diet -- From Cardiovascular Disease." ScienceDaily. Web. ScienceDaily, 20 July 2008. www.sciencedaily.com/releases/2008/07/080718075357.htm.

35. Furey, Matt. "100 Steps to 99 Years." http://theunbeatableman.com/. Web. 26 Aug, 2006. http://theunbeatableman.com/uncensored/uncategorized/100-steps-to-99-years/

36. O'Connor, Anahad. "Really? The Claim: Taking a Walk After a Meal Aids Digestion." Web. 24 June, 2014. http://well.blogs.nytimes.com/2013/06/24/really-the-claim-taking-a-walk-after-a-meal-aids-digestion/?_r=0.

37. Hunt, Susan. "The History of the Ozone Layer." http://www.ozonedepletion.co.uk. Web. 9 Oct. 2015. http://www.ozonedepletion.co.uk/history-ozone-layer.html.

38. "Facts About Sunburn and Skin Cancer." The Skin Cancer Foundation. http://www.skincancer.org Web. 2015.

http://www.skincancer.org/prevention/sunburn/facts-about-sunburn-and-skin-cancer.

39. Moskowitz, Clara. "Fact or Fiction?: Energy Can Neither be Created Nor Destroyed." http://www.scientificamerican.com. Web. 5 Aug., 2014. http://www.scientificamerican.com/article/energy-can-neither-be-created-nor-destroyed/.

40. Greenfield, Ben. "Burning More Fat With Cold." http://www.bengreenfieldfitness.com. Web. Sept, 2012. http://www.bengreenfieldfitness.com/2012/09/burning-more-fat-with-cold.

41. "Do 33% of High School Graduates Never Read Another Book For the Rest of their Lives?" Stack Exchange. Forum Question. Web 14 May, 2012. http://skeptics.stackexchange.com/questions/9446/do-33-of-high-school-graduates-never-read-another-book-for-the-rest-of-their-li.

42. Holtcamp, Wendee. "Obesogens: An Environmental Link to Obesity" http://www.ncbi.nlm.nih.gov 1 Feb., 2012. http://www.ncbi.nlm.nih.gov/pmc/articles/PMC3279464.